Global fertility is now 2.5 children per woman

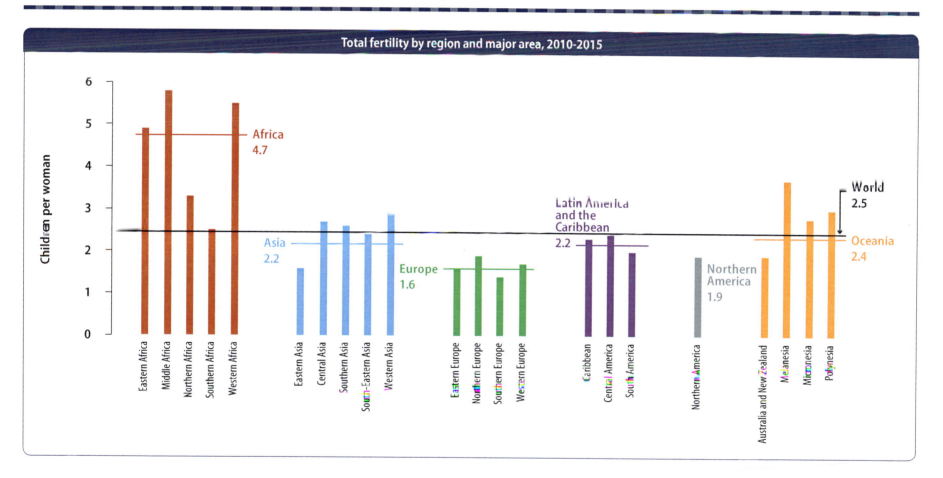

Total fertility by region and major area, 2010-2015

According to the results of the 2015 Revision of World Population Prospects, total fertility is now 2.5 children per woman globally.

This global average masks wide regional differences. Africa remains the region with the highest fertility at 4.7 children per woman. Europe has the lowest fertility of 1.6 children per woman. Both Asia and Latin America and the Caribbean have total fertility of 2.2 children per woman, closely followed by Oceania with 2.4 children per woman.

Middle and Western Africa stand out as having particularly high fertility of over five children per woman. Eastern Asia, Eastern Europe and Southern Europe have very low fertility at under 1.6 children per woman.

Fertility was high in most countries in the world in 1990-1995

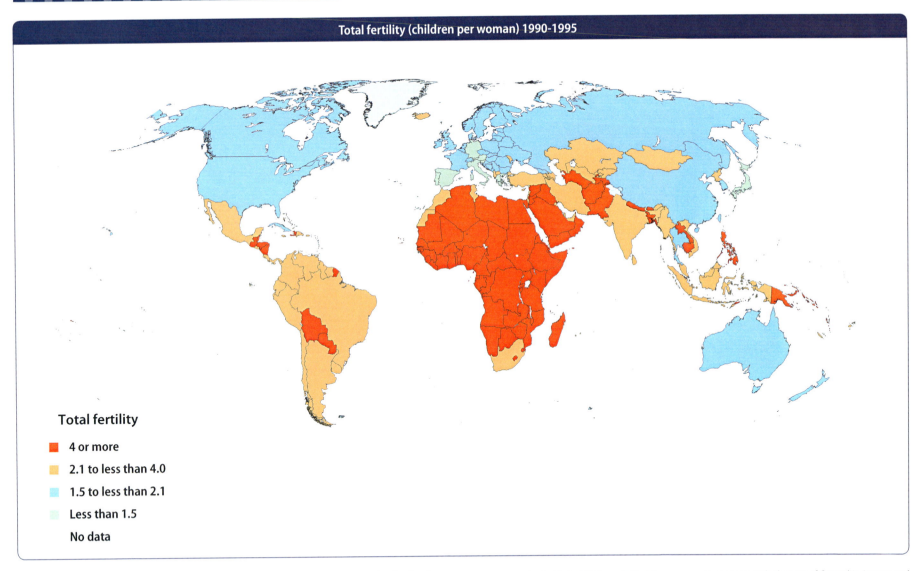

Total fertility (children per woman) 1990-1995

Total fertility

- ■ 4 or more
- ■ 2.1 to less than 4.0
- ■ 1.5 to less than 2.1
- ■ Less than 1.5
- No data

The boundaries and names shown and the designations used on the this map do not imply official endorsement or acceptance by the United Nations. Dotted line represents approximately the Line of Control in Jammu and Kashmir agreeed upon by India and Pakistan. The final status of Jammu and Kashmir has not yet been agreed upon by the parties. Final Boundary between the Republic of Sudan and the Republic of South Sudan has not yet been determined.

Fertility has declined but remains high in sub-Saharan Africa

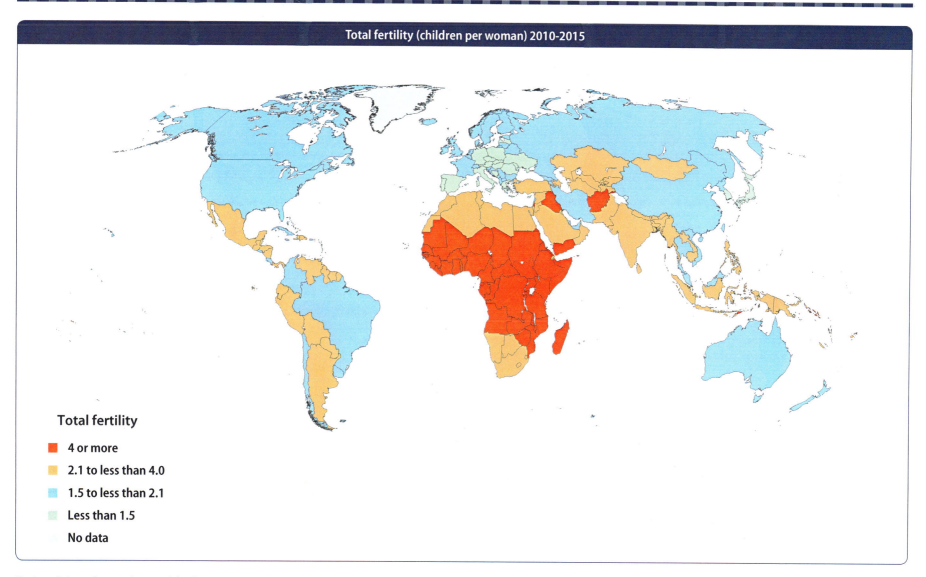

Total fertility (children per woman) 2010-2015

Total fertility

- 4 or more
- 2.1 to less than 4.0
- 1.5 to less than 2.1
- Less than 1.5
- No data

The boundaries and names shown and the designations used on the this map do not imply official endorsement or acceptance by the United Nations. Dotted line represents approximately the Line of Control in Jammu and Kashmir agreeed upon by India and Pakistan. The final status of Jammu and Kashmir has not yet been agreed upon by the parties. Final Boundary between the Republic of Sudan and the Republic of South Sudan has not yet been determined.

Nearly half the world lives in below-replacement level fertility countries

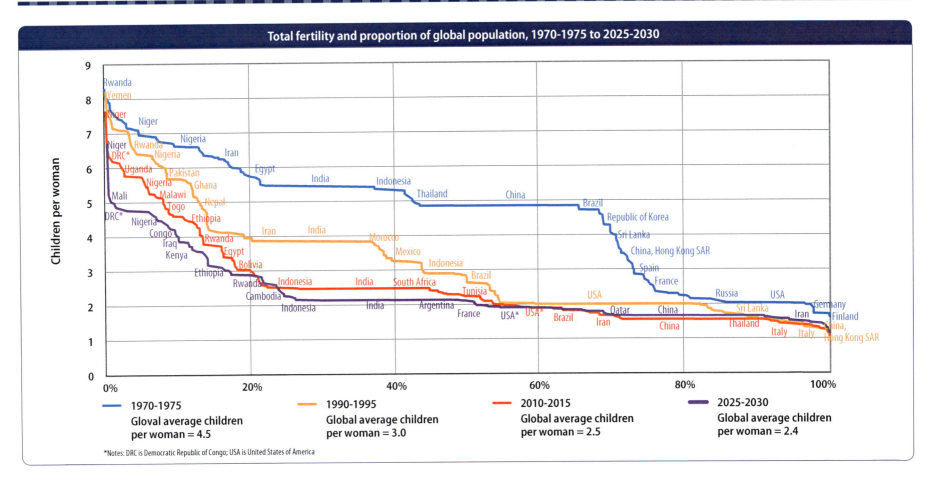

Total fertility and proportion of global population, 1970-1975 to 2025-2030

Legend:
- 1970-1975 — Gloval average children per woman = 4.5
- 1990-1995 — Global average children per woman = 3.0
- 2010-2015 — Global average children per woman = 2.5
- 2025-2030 — Global average children per woman = 2.4

*Notes: DRC is Democratic Republic of Congo; USA is United States of America

Today, 46 per cent of the world's population lives in countries with low levels of fertility, where women have fewer than 2.1 children on average.

Low-fertility countries now include all of Europe and Northern America, as well as many countries in Asia and Latin America and the Caribbean.

Another 46 per cent of the world's population lives in "intermediate-fertility" countries that have already experienced substantial fertility declines and where women have on average between 2.1 and 5 children.

The remaining 8 per cent of the world's population lives in "high-fertility" countries that have experienced only limited fertility decline to date. In these countries the average woman has five or more children over her lifetime. Most of these countries are in sub-Saharan Africa.

Shifts over time in the top ten lowest and highest fertility countries or areas

The increasing concentration of high-fertility countries in one region can be seen in the top ten highest fertility countries or areas. While half were in sub-Saharan Africa in 1970-1975, this increased to eight countries in 1990-1995 and nine countries in 2010-2015.

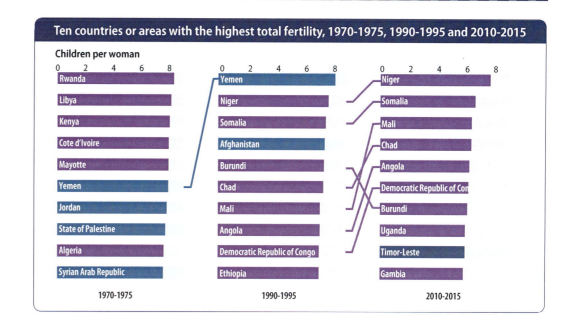

The top ten lowest fertility countries or areas are no longer primarily in Europe. In 1970-1975 eight of the ten countries or areas were in Europe. By 1990-1995, there were three in Asia and by 2010-2015, half of the top ten lowest fertility countries or areas were in Asia.

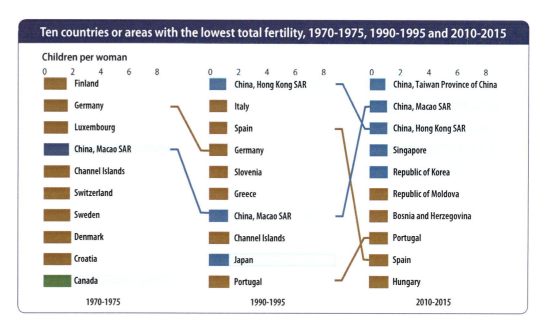

Fertility is projected to decline slowly in Africa

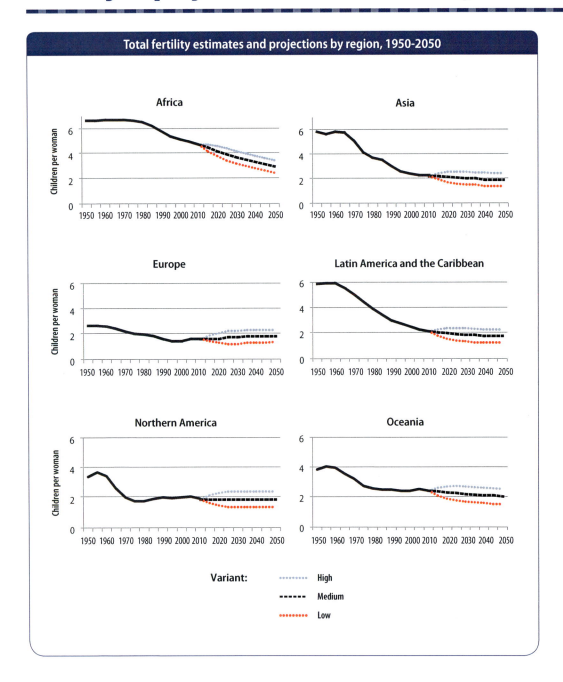

Total fertility estimates and projections by region, 1950-2050

Variant:
- High
- Medium
- Low

Global total fertility is projected to decline to 2.4 children per woman by 2030 and 2.2 children per woman by 2050.

In Africa, fertility is projected to decline to 3.9 children per woman by 2030 and 3.1 children per woman by 2050. Fertility declines in all other regions are projected to be much more modest and even show small increases in Europe and Northern America.

The slower projected pace of fertility decline in Africa compared with the pace experienced by Asia and Latin America and the Caribbean at similar levels of fertility has important population and development implications for Africa.

Sex ratios at birth are imbalanced in some countries, especially in Asia

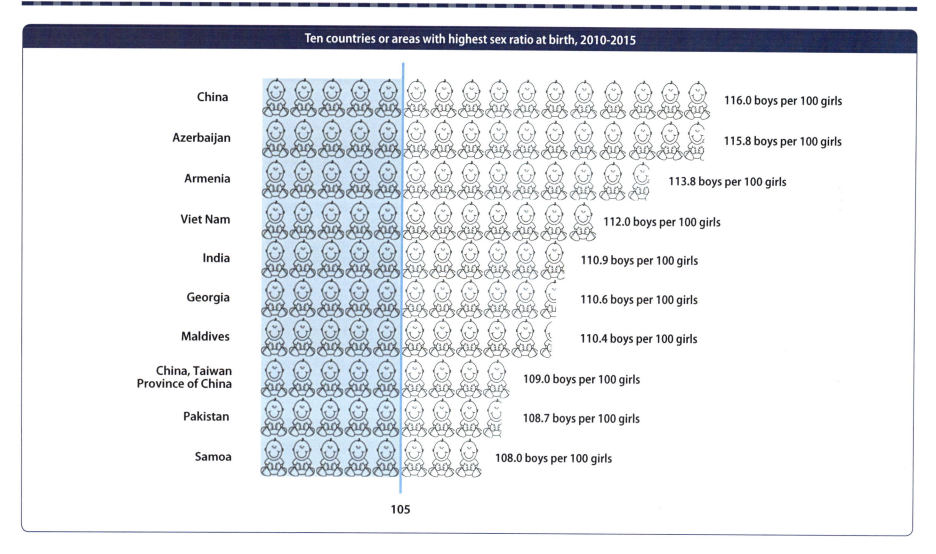

Ten countries or areas with highest sex ratio at birth, 2010-2015

China — 116.0 boys per 100 girls
Azerbaijan — 115.8 boys per 100 girls
Armenia — 113.8 boys per 100 girls
Viet Nam — 112.0 boys per 100 girls
India — 110.9 boys per 100 girls
Georgia — 110.6 boys per 100 girls
Maldives — 110.4 boys per 100 girls
China, Taiwan Province of China — 109.0 boys per 100 girls
Pakistan — 108.7 boys per 100 girls
Samoa — 108.0 boys per 100 girls

105

The standard biological sex ratio at birth is around 104 to 106 boys per 100 girls. Sex ratios above this range indicate the use of practices and methods, including sex-selective abortion, to realize strong preferences for sons.

The current sex ratios among children will have a lasting impact on population dynamics with men of marriageable age already outnumbering women in many countries, especially in Asia which has nine out of the ten countries or areas with the highest sex ratio at birth.

Each woman in the world is replacing herself with just over one surviving daughter on average

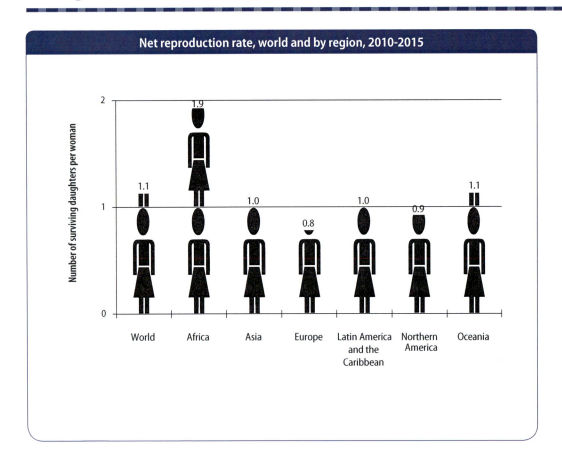

Net reproduction rate, world and by region, 2010-2015

Number of surviving daughters per woman

- World: 1.1
- Africa: 1.9
- Asia: 1.0
- Europe: 0.8
- Latin America and the Caribbean: 1.0
- Northern America: 0.9
- Oceania: 1.1

The net reproduction rate is the average number of daughters that would be born to a woman taking into account the prevailing levels of fertility, female mortality and the sex ratio at birth. When the net reproduction rate is one, each woman is exactly replacing herself with one surviving daughter and this implies that fertility is at replacement level.

Where more boys than expected are born compared with girls, the net reproduction rate will be lower than expected for a given fertility rate and the long-term population growth rate will be lower as a result. This is the case in many countries in Asia.

Globally, the net reproduction rate is 1.1 surviving daughters per woman. In all regions in the world, the net reproduction rate is at or below this level, except for Africa, where the net reproduction rate is 1.9. This means that, on average, each African mother is replacing herself with nearly two daughters, which leads to fast population growth.

Africa remains the region with the highest adolescent birth rate

The adolescent birth rate is the number of births per 1,000 women ages 15 to 19. Early childbearing poses increased health risks to adolescent mothers and reduces the education and employment opportunities that adolescent girls might have had otherwise.

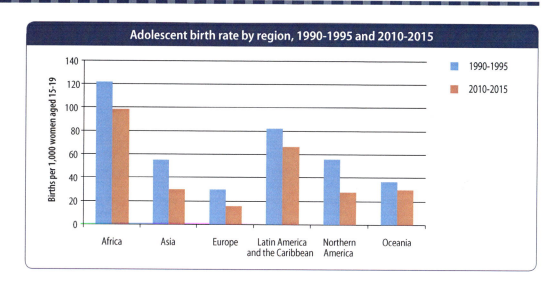

The trend in adolescent fertility has been downward in all regions but there are very sharp differences in levels and trends. Africa has the highest adolescent birth rate and the decline over time has been slow. High adolescent fertility also persists in Latin America and the Caribbean.

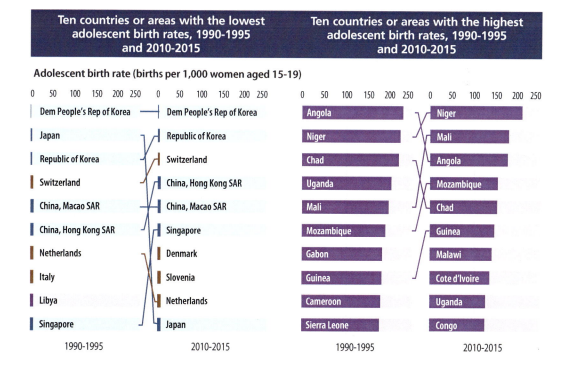

Adolescent birth rates were high in 1990-1995, especially in sub-Saharan Africa

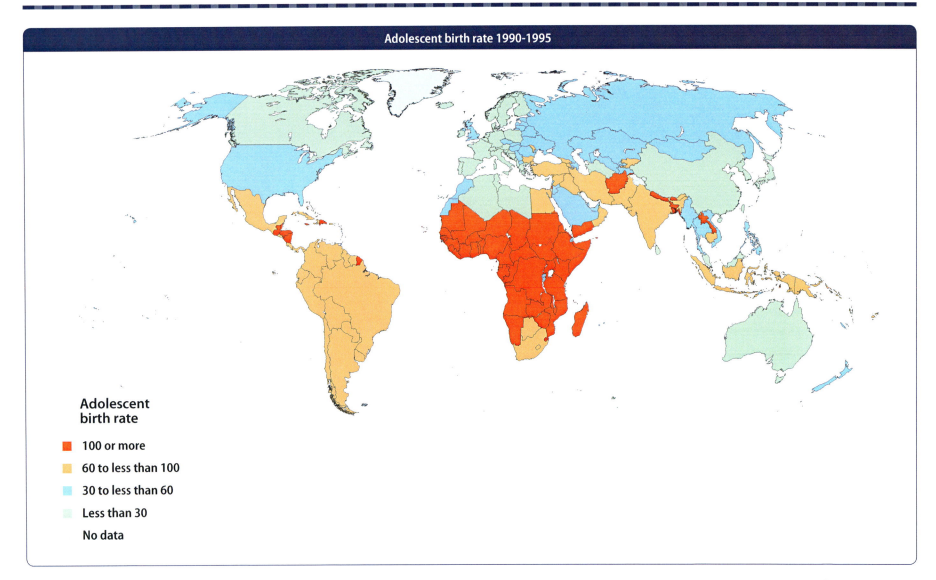

Adolescent birth rate 1990-1995

Adolescent birth rate

- 🟥 100 or more
- 🟧 60 to less than 100
- 🟦 30 to less than 60
- 🟩 Less than 30
- No data

The boundaries and names shown and the designations used on the this map do not imply official endorsement or acceptance by the United Nations. Dotted line represents approximately the Line of Control in Jammu and Kashmir agreeed upon by India and Pakistan. The final status of Jammu and Kashmir has not yet been agreed upon by the parties. Final Boundary between the Republic of Sudan and the Republic of South Sudan has not yet been determined.

Adolescents are having fewer children in most countries of the world

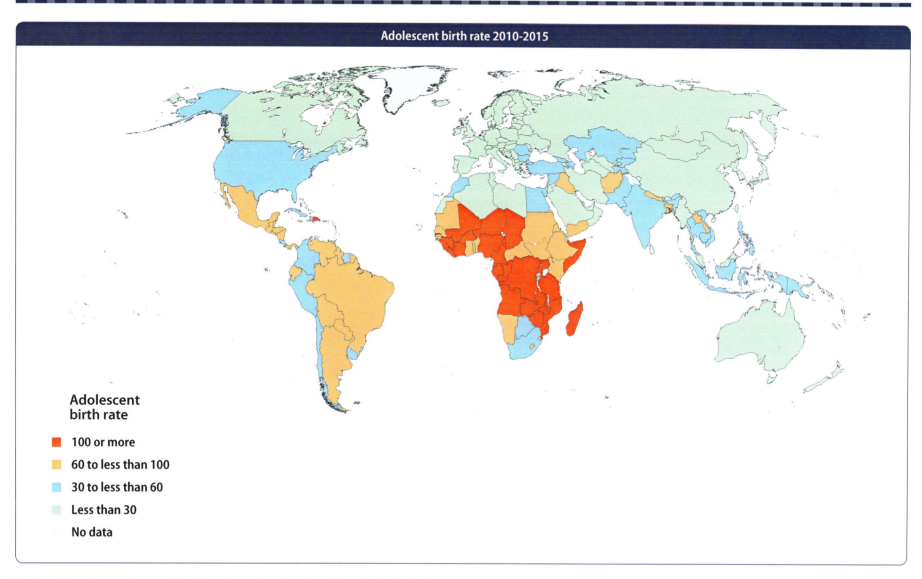

Adolescent birth rate 2010-2015

Adolescent birth rate

- 100 or more
- 60 to less than 100
- 30 to less than 60
- Less than 30
- No data

The boundaries and names shown and the designations used on the this map do not imply official endorsement or acceptance by the United Nations. Dotted line represents approximately the Line of Control in Jammu and Kashmir agreeed upon by India and Pakistan. The final status of Jammu and Kashmir has not yet been agreed upon by the parties. Final Boundary between the Republic of Sudan and the Republic of South Sudan has not yet been determined.

Mean age at childbearing decreased in regions where fertility was declining

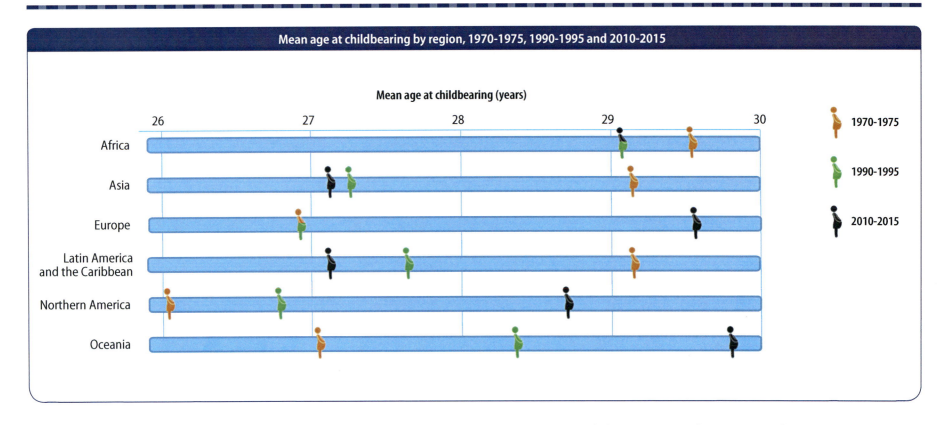

Mean age at childbearing by region, 1970-1975, 1990-1995 and 2010-2015

Mean age at childbearing (years)

In Africa, Asia, and Latin America and the Caribbean, the greater proportional decline of childbearing of women at older ages has led to a decreasing mean age at childbearing.

In Europe and Northern America, where fertility was already relatively low by 1970-1975, the postponement of childbearing has led to an increasing mean age at childbearing.

Countries can differ greatly in the age pattern of childbearing

At higher fertility levels, the differences in how births are distributed by the age of mother between countries are small although there can be relatively large differences in the adolescent birth rate. For example, both Côte d'Ivoire and Afghanistan have a high fertility level of 5.1 children per woman but adolescent childbearing accounts for 13 per cent of births in Côte d'Ivoire and only 9 per cent of births in Afghanistan.

At lower levels of fertility, the differences in the age distribution of births tend to be larger. For example, both India and Libya have total fertility of 2.5 children per woman. However, more than three in four of all births in India are to women under the age of 30 (78 per cent) compared with only about one in three births in Libya (34 per cent).

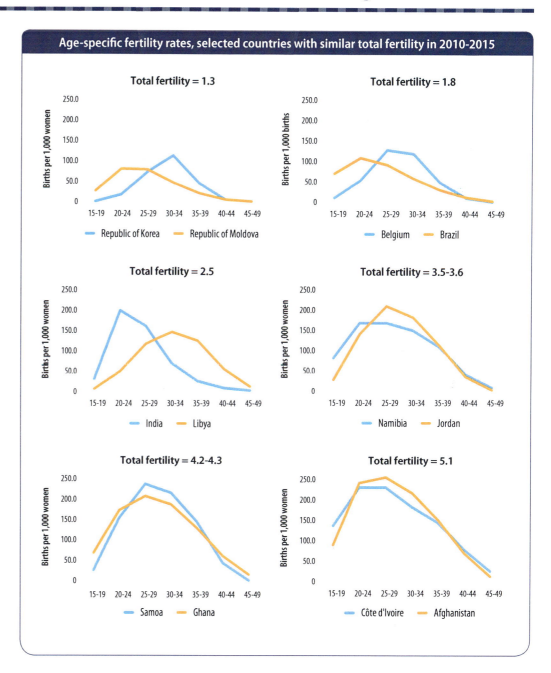

Age-specific fertility rates, selected countries with similar total fertility in 2010-2015

Country or area	Total fertility (children per woman)				Trends	Net reproduction rate	Adolescent birth rate (births per thousand women aged 15-19)				Trends
	1970-1975	1990-1995	2010-2015	2025-2030		2010-2015	1970-1975	1990-1995	2010-2015	2025-2030	
World	**4.5**	**3.0**	**2.5**	**2.4**		**1.1**	**75**	**65**	**46**	**37**	
More developed regions [a]	**2.2**	**1.7**	**1.7**	**1.8**		**0.8**	**39**	**34**	**19**	**9**	
Less developed regions [b]	**5.4**	**3.4**	**2.6**	**2.5**		**1.2**	**85**	**71**	**50**	**40**	
Least developed countries [c]	6.7	5.8	4.3	3.5		1.8	152	133	97	72	
Other less developed countries [d]	5.2	3.1	2.4	2.2		1.0	77	61	39	31	
Less developed regions, excluding China	**5.7**	**4.0**	**3.0**	**2.6**		**1.3**	**110**	**89**	**59**	**46**	
High-income countries [e]	**2.3**	**1.8**	**1.7**	**1.8**		**0.8**	**41**	**34**	**22**	**13**	
Middle-income countries [e]	**5.2**	**3.2**	**2.4**	**2.3**		**1.1**	**81**	**66**	**42**	**33**	
Upper-middle-income countries [e]	4.9	2.4	1.9	1.8		0.8	52	39	30	26	
Lower-middle-income countries [e]	5.6	4.0	2.9	2.5		1.3	113	90	50	37	
Low-income countries [e]	**6.6**	**6.2**	**4.9**	**3.9**		**2.0**	**134**	**133**	**103**	**76**	
Sub-Saharan Africa [f]	**6.8**	**6.2**	**5.1**	**4.1**		**2.1**	**152**	**139**	**109**	**80**	
Africa	**6.7**	**5.7**	**4.7**	**3.9**		**1.9**	**145**	**122**	**98**	**73**	
Eastern Africa	**7.1**	**6.4**	**4.9**	**3.9**		**2.1**	**142**	**134**	**99**	**67**	
Burundi	7.3	7.4	6.1	4.9		2.4	48	49	30	21	
Comoros	7.1	6.1	4.6	3.6		2.0	128	108	74	48	
Djibouti	6.8	5.9	3.3	2.6		1.4	53	45	23	16	
Eritrea	6.6	6.2	4.4	3.4		1.9	115	108	61	35	
Ethiopia	7.1	7.1	4.6	3.1		2.0	119	118	67	33	
Kenya	8.0	5.6	4.4	3.6		1.9	181	114	94	75	
Madagascar	7.3	6.1	4.5	3.7		2.0	163	150	123	91	
Malawi	7.4	6.7	5.3	4.2		2.2	197	164	140	114	
Mauritius [1]	3.5	2.2	1.5	1.5		0.7	56	43	29	26	
Mayotte	7.9	5.3	4.1	3.2		2.0	186	90	62	46	
Mozambique	6.6	6.1	5.5	4.5		2.2	127	189	154	95	
Réunion	3.9	2.4	2.2	2.0		1.1	62	51	42	48	
Rwanda	8.3	6.6	4.1	3.0		1.8	75	59	30	16	
Seychelles	5.4	2.6	2.3	2.0		1.1	146	68	60	47	
Somalia	7.1	7.5	6.6	5.2		2.6	54	102	110	78	
South Sudan	6.9	6.7	5.2	4.0		2.0	148	136	78	34	
Uganda	7.1	7.1	5.9	4.6		2.4	182	201	127	69	
United Republic of Tanzania [2]	6.8	6.1	5.2	4.3		2.3	155	140	123	98	
Zambia	7.4	6.4	5.5	4.6		2.2	189	163	103	56	
Zimbabwe	7.4	4.8	4.0	3.1		1.7	174	111	113	90	
Middle Africa	**6.5**	**6.8**	**5.8**	**4.6**		**2.3**	**180**	**164**	**133**	**98**	
Angola	7.4	7.2	6.2	5.0		2.3	234	227	176	121	
Cameroon	6.3	6.2	4.8	3.8		1.9	190	178	116	70	

Country or area	Share of total fertility by women under age 20 (per cent) 2010-2015	Age-specific fertility rate 2010-2015 (births per thousand women in age group)							Age distribution
		15-19	20-24	25-29	30-34	35-39	40-44	45-49	
World	9	46	149	144	95	48	16	4	
More developed regions [a]	6	19	65	98	93	47	10	1	
Less developed regions [b]	9	50	162	152	95	48	17	5	
Least developed countries [c]	11	97	210	211	163	108	49	16	
Other less developed countries [d]	8	39	153	142	84	40	13	3	
Less developed regions, excluding China	10	59	171	164	110	62	23	7	
High-income countries [e]	6	22	66	101	98	51	11	1	
Middle-income countries [e]	9	42	156	144	84	40	14	4	
Upper-middle-income countries [e]	8	30	126	117	62	26	8	1	
Lower-middle-income countries [e]	9	50	180	166	103	54	20	6	
Low-income countries [e]	11	103	229	241	193	130	61	21	
Sub-Saharan Africa [f]	11	109	230	243	200	142	69	25	
Africa	10	98	216	229	187	131	61	21	
Eastern Africa	10	99	234	242	193	131	64	25	
Burundi	2	30	233	352	285	188	102	24	
Comoros	8	74	182	210	218	139	67	30	
Djibouti	4	23	78	147	187	148	58	18	
Eritrea	7	61	194	220	200	132	58	15	
Ethiopia	7	67	203	224	193	132	68	30	
Kenya	11	94	221	221	163	112	46	31	
Madagascar	14	123	222	222	163	107	51	12	
Malawi	13	140	252	220	190	140	81	27	
Mauritius [1]	10	29	75	92	66	29	7	0	
Mayotte	8	62	183	188	178	132	62	15	
Mozambique	14	154	243	231	197	155	77	33	
Réunion	9	42	98	129	110	54	16	1	
Rwanda	4	30	166	231	182	120	66	13	
Seychelles	13	60	118	133	93	50	11	1	
Somalia	8	110	274	325	258	189	107	59	
South Sudan	8	78	224	279	209	123	75	43	
Uganda	11	127	317	303	221	137	55	24	
United Republic of Tanzania [2]	12	123	262	257	200	131	61	13	
Zambia	9	103	267	265	210	152	72	20	
Zimbabwe	14	113	203	188	149	103	38	9	
Middle Africa	11	133	264	281	227	162	76	20	
Angola	14	176	319	324	223	129	59	10	
Cameroon	12	116	219	244	193	126	49	16	

Country or area	Total fertility (children per woman)				Trends	Net reproduction rate	Adolescent birth rate (births per thousand women aged 15-19)				Trends
	1970-1975	1990-1995	2010-2015	2025-2030		2010-2015	1970-1975	1990-1995	2010-2015	2025-2030	
Middle Africa (continued)											
Central African Republic	6.0	5.7	4.4	3.3		1.6	175	143	98	67	
Chad	6.7	7.4	6.3	4.8		2.3	209	218	152	79	
Congo	6.4	5.2	5.0	4.1		2.1	147	130	125	90	
Dem. Republic of the Congo	6.3	7.1	6.2	4.8		2.5	156	133	124	105	
Equatorial Guinea	5.7	5.9	5.0	3.7		2.0	130	134	114	82	
Gabon	5.2	5.2	4.0	3.2		1.7	201	181	111	66	
São Tomé and Príncipe	6.5	5.7	4.7	3.8		2.1	137	115	89	67	
Northern Africa	**6.4**	**4.2**	**3.3**	**2.8**		**1.5**	**121**	**59**	**47**	**33**	
Algeria	7.6	4.1	2.9	2.3		1.4	103	24	11	8	
Egypt	5.7	4.1	3.4	2.8		1.6	128	80	55	42	
Libya	8.1	4.2	2.5	2.0		1.2	132	8	6	6	
Morocco	6.4	3.7	2.6	2.1		1.2	128	37	33	25	
Sudan	6.9	6.0	4.5	3.6		1.9	152	108	84	46	
Tunisia	6.4	3.0	2.2	1.9		1.0	43	17	7	7	
Western Sahara	6.6	4.0	2.2	1.8		1.0	131	59	23	14	
Southern Africa	**5.6**	**3.5**	**2.5**	**2.2**		**1.1**	**82**	**92**	**54**	**34**	
Botswana	6.5	4.3	2.9	2.3		1.3	158	85	39	17	
Lesotho	5.8	4.7	3.3	2.6		1.3	82	86	90	90	
Namibia	6.6	4.9	3.6	2.9		1.6	139	103	80	63	
South Africa	5.5	3.3	2.4	2.1		1.0	76	91	51	31	
Swaziland	6.9	5.3	3.4	2.6		1.3	151	125	86	39	
Western Africa	**6.8**	**6.4**	**5.5**	**4.6**		**2.1**	**171**	**146**	**120**	**93**	
Benin	6.8	6.6	4.9	3.8		2.0	93	127	90	59	
Burkina Faso	6.7	6.9	5.6	4.5		2.3	169	145	115	82	
Cabo Verde	6.9	4.9	2.4	1.9		1.1	116	109	75	63	
Côte d'Ivoire	7.9	6.4	5.1	4.2		1.9	217	148	135	125	
Gambia	6.2	6.1	5.8	4.9		2.4	216	153	116	95	
Ghana	6.9	5.3	4.2	3.5		1.8	142	104	70	53	
Guinea	6.3	6.5	5.1	4.0		2.1	181	180	146	114	
Guinea-Bissau	6.1	6.5	5.0	3.9		1.9	108	138	99	59	
Liberia	6.8	6.3	4.8	3.9		2.0	214	161	117	79	
Mali	7.2	7.2	6.4	5.0		2.5	194	196	179	145	
Mauritania	6.7	5.9	4.7	3.9		2.0	121	106	82	63	
Niger	7.5	7.7	7.6	6.7		3.1	214	222	208	168	
Nigeria	6.6	6.4	5.7	4.7		2.1	168	143	117	86	
Senegal	7.4	6.3	5.2	4.2		2.3	188	126	87	53	
Sierra Leone	6.1	6.6	4.8	3.4		1.8	191	176	125	86	
Togo	7.2	6.0	4.7	3.8		2.0	145	110	92	84	

Country or area	Share of total fertility by women under age 20 (per cent) 2010-2015	Age-specific fertility rate 2010-2015 (births per thousand women in age group)							Age distribution
		15-19	20-24	25-29	30-34	35-39	40-44	45-49	
Middle Africa (continued)									
Central African Republic	11	98	191	202	161	113	61	55	
Chad	12	152	324	321	252	147	54	13	
Congo	13	125	244	232	186	125	60	18	
Dem. Republic of the Congo	10	124	260	285	247	195	96	23	
Equatorial Guinea	12	114	242	249	155	122	76	35	
Gabon	14	111	166	182	165	113	55	8	
São Tomé and Príncipe	9	89	202	200	191	162	83	8	
Northern Africa	**7**	**47**	**155**	**176**	**141**	**92**	**34**	**9**	
Algeria	2	11	92	151	147	125	52	7	
Egypt	8	55	208	195	131	67	17	4	
Libya	1	6	48	116	146	124	55	11	
Morocco	7	33	99	123	118	85	41	13	
Sudan	9	84	192	243	190	112	50	21	
Tunisia	2	7	57	123	132	88	23	2	
Western Sahara	5	23	78	108	104	77	38	13	
Southern Africa	**11**	**54**	**134**	**136**	**95**	**57**	**22**	**6**	
Botswana	7	39	138	137	117	90	45	14	
Lesotho	14	90	175	146	112	78	44	6	
Namibia	11	80	167	168	149	108	41	9	
South Africa	11	51	129	133	90	52	19	6	
Swaziland	13	86	177	164	127	78	28	12	
Western Africa	**11**	**120**	**232**	**254**	**222**	**166**	**83**	**31**	
Benin	9	90	226	256	204	126	56	19	
Burkina Faso	10	115	249	265	226	168	83	23	
Cabo Verde	16	75	120	119	78	51	28	3	
Côte d'Ivoire	13	135	229	230	182	142	77	25	
Gambia	10	116	244	268	235	168	83	42	
Ghana	8	70	174	208	187	130	63	19	
Guinea	14	146	209	225	201	142	76	28	
Guinea-Bissau	10	99	211	248	203	144	62	23	
Liberia	12	117	217	229	188	129	65	21	
Mali	14	179	264	284	240	173	92	38	
Mauritania	9	82	171	211	201	159	83	31	
Niger	14	208	334	326	287	220	102	49	
Nigeria	10	117	235	260	232	178	91	35	
Senegal	8	87	209	244	225	172	81	18	
Sierra Leone	13	125	212	216	178	132	65	30	
Togo	10	92	210	240	182	133	64	17	

Country or area	Total fertility (children per woman)				Trends	Net reproduction rate	Adolescent birth rate (births per thousand women aged 15-19)				Trends
	1970-1975	1990-1995	2010-2015	2025-2030		2010-2015	1970-1975	1990-1995	2010-2015	2025-2030	
Asia	**5.1**	**3.0**	**2.2**	**2.0**		**1.0**	**70**	**56**	**30**	**22**	
Eastern Asia	**4.4**	**2.0**	**1.6**	**1.6**		**0.7**	**27**	**16**	**7**	**6**	
China [3]	4.9	2.0	1.6	1.7		0.7	30	17	8	7	
China, Hong Kong SAR [4]	3.3	1.2	1.2	1.4		0.6	18	7	4	3	
China, Macao SAR [5]	1.8	1.4	1.2	1.5		0.6	6	7	4	3	
China, Taiwan Province of China	3.4	1.8	1.1	1.2		0.5	37	17	4	1	
Dem. People's Rep. of Korea	4.0	2.3	2.0	1.9		0.9	4	2	1	0	
Japan	2.1	1.5	1.4	1.6		0.7	5	4	5	3	
Mongolia	7.5	3.3	2.7	2.3		1.3	83	38	19	8	
Republic of Korea	4.3	1.7	1.3	1.4		0.6	14	4	2	1	
South-Central Asia [6]	**5.6**	**4.0**	**2.6**	**2.2**		**1.1**	**114**	**95**	**38**	**21**	
Central Asia	**4.8**	**3.5**	**2.7**	**2.3**		**1.2**	**39**	**55**	**26**	**20**	
Kazakhstan	3.5	2.6	2.6	2.3		1.2	33	54	31	19	
Kyrgyzstan	4.7	3.6	3.1	2.6		1.5	43	68	42	32	
Tajikistan	6.8	4.9	3.6	2.9		1.6	65	57	39	32	
Turkmenistan	6.2	4.0	2.3	2.0		1.1	30	26	18	12	
Uzbekistan	5.7	3.8	2.5	2.1		1.1	38	58	18	15	
Southern Asia	**5.7**	**4.0**	**2.6**	**2.2**		**1.1**	**118**	**97**	**39**	**21**	
Afghanistan	7.5	7.5	5.1	3.0		2.1	145	164	88	36	
Bangladesh	6.9	4.1	2.2	1.8		1.0	204	143	85	69	
Bhutan	6.7	5.1	2.1	1.7		1.0	110	102	28	9	
India	5.4	3.8	2.5	2.1		1.1	109	94	30	12	
Iran (Islamic Republic of)	6.2	4.0	1.7	1.5		0.8	136	75	29	20	
Maldives	7.2	5.2	2.2	1.7		1.0	212	103	9	2	
Nepal	5.9	5.0	2.3	1.8		1.1	130	135	75	58	
Pakistan	6.6	5.7	3.7	2.9		1.6	110	76	41	30	
Sri Lanka	4.0	2.4	2.1	1.9		1.0	49	29	18	8	
South-eastern Asia	**5.5**	**3.1**	**2.4**	**2.1**		**1.1**	**84**	**51**	**44**	**43**	
Brunei Darussalam	5.9	3.3	1.9	1.7		0.9	55	44	22	18	
Cambodia	6.2	5.1	2.7	2.3		1.2	90	67	49	54	
Indonesia	5.3	2.9	2.5	2.1		1.2	129	63	52	41	
Lao People's Dem. Republic	6.0	5.9	3.1	2.3		1.4	105	105	66	52	
Malaysia [7]	4.6	3.4	2.0	1.8		0.9	48	19	13	15	
Myanmar	5.7	3.2	2.3	2.0		1.0	91	31	18	13	
Philippines	6.0	4.1	3.0	2.6		1.4	56	51	57	69	
Singapore	2.8	1.7	1.2	1.3		0.6	25	8	4	4	
Thailand	5.1	2.0	1.5	1.4		0.7	61	50	45	41	
Timor-Leste	5.5	5.7	5.9	4.3		2.7	58	59	52	29	

Country or area	Share of total fertility by women under age 20 (per cent) 2010-2015	Age-specific fertility rate 2010-2015 (births per thousand women in age group)							Age distribution
		15-19	20-24	25-29	30-34	35-39	40-44	45-49	
Asia	**7**	**30**	**151**	**138**	**76**	**32**	**10**	**2**	
Eastern Asia	**2**	**7**	**123**	**111**	**49**	**15**	**4**	**1**	
China [3]	2	8	134	113	40	11	4	1	
China, Hong Kong SAR [4]	1	4	24	57	95	52	9	0	
China, Macao SAR [5]	1	4	40	77	65	39	14	0	
China, Taiwan Province of China	2	4	23	65	81	36	5	0	
Dem. People's Rep. of Korea	0	1	58	209	110	18	3	0	
Japan	2	5	34	87	97	48	9	0	
Mongolia	4	19	142	164	110	69	28	3	
Republic of Korea	1	2	17	71	112	44	4	0	
South-Central Asia [6]	**7**	**38**	**185**	**159**	**83**	**34**	**11**	**3**	
Central Asia	**5**	**26**	**176**	**170**	**107**	**47**	**13**	**1**	
Kazakhstan	6	31	153	156	109	62	16	1	
Kyrgyzstan	7	42	189	175	124	70	22	3	
Tajikistan	6	39	216	217	145	69	22	1	
Turkmenistan	4	18	129	166	106	42	7	1	
Uzbekistan	4	18	182	165	94	29	7	1	
Southern Asia	**8**	**39**	**185**	**158**	**82**	**34**	**11**	**4**	
Afghanistan	9	88	240	254	215	149	68	12	
Bangladesh	19	85	150	113	62	25	8	3	
Bhutan	7	28	112	125	86	44	21	4	
India	6	30	199	159	69	26	9	3	
Iran (Islamic Republic of)	8	29	81	103	86	39	9	2	
Maldives	2	9	120	140	108	48	11	1	
Nepal	16	75	174	110	55	30	15	3	
Pakistan	5	41	182	224	174	85	29	9	
Sri Lanka	4	18	69	141	120	57	16	2	
South-eastern Asia	**9**	**44**	**120**	**128**	**99**	**57**	**19**	**4**	
Brunei Darussalam	6	22	79	117	90	56	16	1	
Cambodia	9	49	163	152	103	51	17	4	
Indonesia	10	52	130	132	103	59	18	5	
Lao People's Dem. Republic	11	66	170	178	112	68	22	4	
Malaysia [7]	3	13	55	117	118	70	21	2	
Myanmar	4	18	83	119	114	81	31	5	
Philippines	9	57	148	147	127	84	37	7	
Singapore	2	4	20	74	95	46	8	0	
Thailand	15	45	81	82	63	29	7	0	
Timor-Leste	4	52	241	307	272	186	88	36	

Country or area	Total fertility (children per woman)				Trends	Net reproduction rate	Adolescent birth rate (births per thousand women aged 15-19)				Trends
	1970-1975	1990-1995	2010-2015	2025-2030		2010-2015	1970-1975	1990-1995	2010-2015	2025-2030	
South-eastern Asia (continued)											
Viet Nam	6.3	3.2	2.0	1.9		0.9	19	34	36	40	
Western Asia	**5.7**	**4.0**	**2.9**	**2.5**		**1.4**	**107**	**67**	**42**	**36**	
Armenia	3.0	2.4	1.6	1.5		0.7	41	80	26	17	
Azerbaijan [8]	4.3	2.9	2.3	2.1		1.0	29	38	54	71	
Bahrain	5.9	3.4	2.1	1.8		1.0	74	22	14	12	
Cyprus [9]	2.5	2.3	1.5	1.5		0.7	21	24	5	4	
Georgia [10]	2.6	2.1	1.8	1.8		0.8	87	69	47	14	
Iraq	7.2	5.6	4.6	3.9		2.1	121	67	80	88	
Israel	3.8	2.9	3.1	2.7		1.5	43	19	12	5	
Jordan	7.8	5.1	3.5	2.7		1.7	100	49	26	15	
Kuwait	7.0	2.4	2.2	1.9		1.0	143	21	12	6	
Lebanon	4.7	2.8	1.7	1.7		0.8	69	39	14	10	
Oman	7.4	6.3	2.9	2.1		1.4	137	73	11	3	
Qatar	6.8	3.7	2.1	1.8		1.0	89	44	12	8	
Saudi Arabia	7.3	5.6	2.9	2.2		1.4	125	60	11	4	
State of Palestine [11]	7.7	6.6	4.3	3.4		2.0	111	110	61	47	
Syrian Arab Republic	7.5	4.8	3.0	2.4		1.4	118	68	42	29	
Turkey	5.3	2.9	2.1	1.9		1.0	113	61	32	17	
United Arab Emirates	6.4	3.9	1.8	1.6		0.9	163	42	28	32	
Yemen	7.9	8.2	4.4	3.0		1.9	169	146	65	45	
Europe	**2.2**	**1.6**	**1.6**	**1.7**		**0.8**	**36**	**31**	**16**	**10**	
Eastern Europe	**2.1**	**1.6**	**1.6**	**1.7**		**0.7**	**37**	**49**	**25**	**15**	
Belarus	2.3	1.7	1.6	1.7		0.8	21	44	21	11	
Bulgaria	2.2	1.6	1.5	1.7		0.7	71	67	42	24	
Czech Republic	2.2	1.6	1.5	1.7		0.7	50	41	11	8	
Hungary	2.1	1.7	1.3	1.5		0.6	56	37	19	14	
Poland	2.2	1.9	1.4	1.4		0.7	26	29	15	11	
Republic of Moldova [12]	2.6	2.1	1.3	1.3		0.6	33	63	26	16	
Romania	2.7	1.5	1.5	1.6		0.7	64	48	37	25	
Russian Federation	2.0	1.5	1.7	1.8		0.8	32	52	27	15	
Slovakia	2.5	1.9	1.4	1.5		0.7	41	45	21	16	
Ukraine [13]	2.1	1.6	1.5	1.7		0.7	39	58	28	15	
Northern Europe	**2.1**	**1.8**	**1.9**	**1.9**		**0.9**	**38**	**26**	**14**	**7**	
Channel Islands [14]	1.9	1.5	1.5	1.5		0.7	21	17	8	5	
Denmark	2.0	1.7	1.7	1.8		0.8	28	9	4	4	
Estonia	2.2	1.6	1.6	1.7		0.8	34	47	16	8	
Finland [15]	1.6	1.8	1.7	1.8		0.8	28	11	7	6	

Country or area	Share of total fertility by women under age 20 (per cent) 2010-2015	Age-specific fertility rate 2010-2015 (births per thousand women in age group)							Age distribution
		15-19	20-24	25-29	30-34	35-39	40-44	45-49	
South-eastern Asia (continued)									
Viet Nam	9	36	120	127	72	30	7	1	
Western Asia	**7**	**42**	**136**	**166**	**125**	**76**	**28**	**7**	
Armenia	8	26	119	96	49	17	3	0	
Azerbaijan [8]	12	54	179	133	62	27	5	1	
Bahrain	3	14	91	116	90	68	31	9	
Cyprus [9]	2	5	49	106	91	35	6	1	
Georgia [10]	13	47	117	106	59	25	8	0	
Iraq	9	80	210	240	210	130	50	8	
Israel	2	12	109	175	179	105	29	3	
Jordan	4	26	139	209	180	111	34	3	
Kuwait	3	12	97	121	108	66	24	3	
Lebanon	4	14	64	110	96	43	11	5	
Oman	2	11	96	165	153	98	42	10	
Qatar	3	12	100	107	101	67	25	4	
Saudi Arabia	2	11	67	175	131	108	53	25	
State of Palestine [11]	7	61	217	223	186	120	46	3	
Syrian Arab Republic	7	42	131	161	140	91	34	7	
Turkey	8	32	114	137	85	40	11	2	
United Arab Emirates	8	28	100	140	67	22	2	6	
Yemen	8	65	188	207	175	138	68	28	
Europe	**5**	**16**	**62**	**96**	**90**	**46**	**10**	**1**	
Eastern Europe	**8**	**25**	**80**	**98**	**70**	**32**	**6**	**0**	
Belarus	7	21	90	107	68	26	4	0	
Bulgaria	14	42	72	91	67	27	4	0	
Czech Republic	4	11	42	93	99	38	6	0	
Hungary	7	19	42	78	81	39	7	0	
Poland	5	15	53	94	73	33	7	0	
Republic of Moldova [12]	10	26	80	78	46	20	4	0	
Romania	13	37	71	89	66	28	5	0	
Russian Federation	8	27	89	104	72	34	7	0	
Slovakia	8	21	51	85	78	32	6	0	
Ukraine [13]	9	28	91	90	59	25	5	0	
Northern Europe	**4**	**14**	**59**	**106**	**116**	**64**	**13**	**1**	
Channel Islands [14]	3	8	36	93	102	46	7	0	
Denmark	1	4	37	113	125	55	10	1	
Estonia	5	16	58	100	87	47	10	0	
Finland [15]	2	7	52	107	112	58	12	1	

Country or area	Total fertility (children per woman)				Trends	Net reproduction rate	Adolescent birth rate (births per thousand women aged 15-19)				Trends
	1970-1975	1990-1995	2010-2015	2025-2030		2010-2015	1970-1975	1990-1995	2010-2015	2025-2030	
Northern Europe (continued)											
Iceland	2.9	2.2	2.0	1.8		1.0	71	26	8	2	
Ireland	3.8	1.9	2.0	2.0		1.0	22	16	12	9	
Latvia	2.0	1.6	1.5	1.7		0.7	39	44	15	10	
Lithuania	2.3	1.8	1.6	1.7		0.8	23	45	14	6	
Norway [16]	2.2	1.9	1.8	1.8		0.9	32	16	6	6	
Sweden	1.9	2.0	1.9	1.9		0.9	33	11	5	6	
United Kingdom	2.0	1.8	1.9	1.9		0.9	43	31	18	8	
Southern Europe	**2.5**	**1.4**	**1.4**	**1.5**		**0.7**	**32**	**14**	**10**	**7**	
Albania	4.6	2.8	1.8	1.8		0.8	29	19	21	21	
Bosnia and Herzegovina	2.7	1.7	1.3	1.3		0.6	51	25	11	4	
Croatia	2.0	1.5	1.5	1.5		0.7	53	21	11	6	
Greece	2.3	1.4	1.3	1.4		0.6	39	17	9	5	
Italy	2.3	1.3	1.4	1.6		0.7	30	8	6	5	
Malta	2.0	2.0	1.4	1.6		0.7	13	12	18	13	
Montenegro	2.6	2.0	1.7	1.6		0.8	33	26	13	10	
Portugal	2.8	1.5	1.3	1.3		0.6	32	22	12	6	
Serbia [17]	2.4	2.0	1.6	1.6		0.8	65	36	21	14	
Slovenia	2.2	1.3	1.6	1.7		0.8	56	20	4	3	
Spain [18]	2.9	1.3	1.3	1.5		0.6	17	10	9	7	
TFYR Macedonia [19]	2.9	2.1	1.5	1.6		0.7	46	43	19	14	
Western Europe	**2.0**	**1.5**	**1.7**	**1.8**		**0.8**	**38**	**13**	**8**	**6**	
Austria	2.0	1.5	1.5	1.6		0.7	55	20	9	4	
Belgium	2.0	1.6	1.8	1.9		0.9	31	11	9	7	
France	2.3	1.7	2.0	2.0		1.0	38	11	10	8	
Germany	1.7	1.3	1.4	1.5		0.7	42	16	8	4	
Luxembourg	1.7	1.7	1.6	1.7		0.8	27	13	7	4	
Netherlands	2.1	1.6	1.8	1.8		0.8	19	7	4	4	
Switzerland	1.9	1.5	1.5	1.7		0.7	20	7	3	2	
Latin America and the Caribbean	**5.0**	**3.0**	**2.2**	**1.9**		**1.0**	**95**	**83**	**67**	**53**	
Caribbean	**4.4**	**2.8**	**2.3**	**2.0**		**1.0**	**115**	**82**	**60**	**47**	
Antigua and Barbuda	3.3	2.1	2.1	1.9		1.0	94	66	49	32	
Aruba	2.7	2.2	1.7	1.6		0.8	60	49	27	13	
Bahamas	3.5	2.6	1.9	1.8		0.9	85	70	34	18	
Barbados	2.7	1.7	1.8	1.8		0.9	92	58	47	15	
Cuba	3.6	1.7	1.6	1.6		0.8	143	69	48	36	
Curaçao	2.9	2.3	2.1	2.0		1.0	65	52	35	29	

Country or area	Share of total fertility by women under age 20 (per cent)	Age-specific fertility rate 2010-2015 (births per thousand women in age group)							Age distribution
	2010-2015	15-19	20-24	25-29	30-34	35-39	40-44	45-49	
Northern Europe (continued)									
Iceland	2	8	58	121	126	65	14	1	
Ireland	3	12	51	88	130	98	22	1	
Latvia	5	15	57	94	79	40	10	1	
Lithuania	4	14	55	117	86	34	6	0	
Norway [16]	2	6	49	115	122	57	10	1	
Sweden	1	5	48	114	134	68	14	1	
United Kingdom	5	18	65	105	115	65	14	1	
Southern Europe	**3**	**10**	**40**	**74**	**91**	**55**	**13**	**1**	
Albania	6	21	107	127	72	24	4	1	
Bosnia and Herzegovina	4	11	52	92	70	26	4	0	
Croatia	4	11	55	99	91	40	7	0	
Greece	3	9	33	76	92	48	10	1	
Italy	2	6	33	73	95	61	15	1	
Malta	6	18	39	87	93	43	7	0	
Montenegro	4	13	75	115	90	39	10	1	
Portugal	5	12	38	71	83	43	9	1	
Serbia [17]	7	21	68	99	83	35	6	1	
Slovenia	1	4	44	108	107	44	7	0	
Spain [18]	3	9	29	58	91	62	14	1	
TFYR Macedonia [19]	6	19	72	103	76	28	4	0	
Western Europe	**2**	**8**	**45**	**103**	**111**	**54**	**10**	**1**	
Austria	3	9	44	89	95	47	9	1	
Belgium	2	9	53	127	117	48	9	0	
France	2	10	59	132	127	58	13	1	
Germany	3	8	36	79	95	51	9	0	
Luxembourg	2	7	41	84	110	57	12	1	
Netherlands	1	4	35	108	137	56	9	0	
Switzerland	1	3	32	82	112	63	12	1	
Latin America and the Caribbean	**15**	**67**	**119**	**109**	**76**	**43**	**14**	**3**	
Caribbean	**13**	**60**	**125**	**118**	**89**	**47**	**14**	**4**	
Antigua and Barbuda	12	49	105	124	89	42	9	1	
Aruba	8	27	82	105	80	36	6	0	
Bahamas	9	34	84	99	88	60	11	1	
Barbados	13	47	87	81	73	52	16	2	
Cuba	15	48	100	90	58	24	5	0	
Curaçao	8	35	104	117	98	52	13	1	

Country or area	Total fertility (children per woman)				Trends	Net reproduction rate	Adolescent birth rate (births per thousand women aged 15-19)				Trends
	1970-1975	1990-1995	2010-2015	2025-2030		2010-2015	1970-1975	1990-1995	2010-2015	2025-2030	
Caribbean (continued)											
Dominican Republic	5.7	3.3	2.5	2.1		1.2	131	114	101	82	
Grenada	4.6	3.5	2.2	1.9		1.0	108	83	35	18	
Guadeloupe [20]	4.5	2.1	2.2	2.0		1.1	64	26	17	11	
Haiti	5.6	5.1	3.1	2.5		1.3	64	70	41	31	
Jamaica	5.0	2.8	2.1	1.9		1.0	182	103	64	45	
Martinique	4.1	2.0	2.0	1.8		0.9	55	29	21	14	
Puerto Rico	3.0	2.2	1.6	1.6		0.8	80	73	47	28	
Saint Lucia	5.7	3.2	1.9	1.7		0.9	158	95	56	44	
Saint Vincent and the Grenadines	5.5	2.9	2.0	1.7		1.0	164	88	55	39	
Trinidad and Tobago	3.5	2.2	1.8	1.7		0.8	92	56	35	21	
United States Virgin Islands	4.7	2.8	2.3	2.0		1.1	166	77	47	32	
Central America	**6.5**	**3.5**	**2.4**	**2.0**		**1.1**	**124**	**89**	**69**	**53**	
Belize	6.3	4.3	2.6	2.2		1.3	175	122	70	51	
Costa Rica	4.1	3.0	1.9	1.7		0.9	97	92	59	46	
El Salvador	5.9	3.7	2.0	1.7		0.9	135	99	67	55	
Guatemala	6.2	5.2	3.3	2.6		1.5	138	121	84	66	
Honduras	7.1	4.9	2.5	2.0		1.1	151	126	68	51	
Mexico	6.7	3.3	2.3	1.9		1.1	120	80	66	50	
Nicaragua	6.8	4.2	2.3	1.9		1.1	158	146	93	71	
Panama	4.9	2.9	2.5	2.2		1.2	133	92	79	59	
South America	**4.6**	**2.9**	**2.0**	**1.8**		**1.0**	**81**	**80**	**66**	**53**	
Argentina	3.1	2.9	2.3	2.1		1.1	68	73	64	59	
Bolivia (Plurinational State of)	6.2	4.7	3.0	2.5		1.3	95	91	73	61	
Brazil	4.7	2.6	1.8	1.7		0.9	75	80	68	57	
Chile	3.6	2.4	1.8	1.7		0.9	85	64	49	40	
Colombia	4.9	2.8	1.9	1.7		0.9	88	83	58	31	
Ecuador	5.8	3.6	2.6	2.2		1.2	115	85	77	65	
French Guiana	4.2	4.1	3.5	3.0		1.7	114	105	83	47	
Guyana	5.0	3.4	2.6	2.3		1.2	116	99	90	76	
Paraguay	5.4	4.3	2.6	2.2		1.2	94	92	60	46	
Peru	6.0	3.6	2.5	2.1		1.2	86	70	52	38	
Suriname	5.3	3.2	2.4	2.1		1.1	113	65	48	38	
Uruguay	3.0	2.5	2.0	1.9		1.0	65	71	58	48	
Venezuela (Bolivarian Republic of)	4.9	3.3	2.4	2.1		1.1	107	95	81	68	

Country or area	Share of total fertility by women under age 20 (per cent) 2010-2015	Age-specific fertility rate 2010-2015 (births per thousand women in age group)							Age distribution
		15-19	20-24	25-29	30-34	35-39	40-44	45-49	
Caribbean (continued)									
Dominican Republic	20	101	156	122	82	34	9	2	
Grenada	8	35	97	133	102	53	15	1	
Guadeloupe [20]	4	17	78	122	129	69	17	2	
Haiti	7	41	131	151	136	101	47	17	
Jamaica	15	64	128	106	69	36	12	2	
Martinique	5	21	71	107	104	66	20	1	
Puerto Rico	14	47	96	93	62	25	5	0	
Saint Lucia	15	56	92	96	77	46	17	0	
Saint Vincent and the Grenadines	14	55	106	114	78	38	9	0	
Trinidad and Tobago	10	35	101	101	76	36	10	1	
United States Virgin Islands	10	47	152	124	84	40	9	4	
Central America	**15**	**69**	**130**	**127**	**86**	**47**	**12**	**2**	
Belize	13	70	151	142	99	49	16	1	
Costa Rica	16	59	101	87	70	41	11	1	
El Salvador	17	67	108	98	71	37	13	2	
Guatemala	13	84	173	159	124	80	33	6	
Honduras	14	68	135	114	87	56	28	5	
Mexico	14	66	126	128	83	44	9	2	
Nicaragua	20	93	123	109	76	43	16	5	
Panama	16	79	149	132	88	38	9	1	
South America	**16**	**66**	**113**	**101**	**72**	**41**	**15**	**2**	
Argentina	14	64	109	110	103	63	19	2	
Bolivia (Plurinational State of)	12	73	147	149	115	81	36	8	
Brazil	19	68	108	91	56	29	10	2	
Chile	14	49	85	93	74	42	12	1	
Colombia	15	58	112	97	65	38	15	3	
Ecuador	15	77	139	125	91	55	24	6	
French Guiana	12	83	156	182	151	89	33	3	
Guyana	17	90	156	119	87	50	13	5	
Paraguay	12	60	130	130	103	65	26	5	
Peru	10	52	117	123	106	68	29	5	
Suriname	10	48	117	129	101	59	24	2	
Uruguay	14	58	98	106	86	46	14	1	
Venezuela (Bolivarian Republic of)	17	81	132	119	86	46	15	2	

Country or area	Total fertility (children per woman)				Trends	Net reproduction rate	Adolescent birth rate (births per thousand women aged 15-19)				Trends
	1970-1975	1990-1995	2010-2015	2025-2030		2010-2015	1970-1975	1990-1995	2010-2015	2025-2030	
Northern America	**2.0**	**2.0**	**1.9**	**1.9**		**0.9**	**59**	**56**	**28**	**8**	
Canada	2.0	1.7	1.6	1.6		0.8	37	25	11	7	
United States of America	2.0	2.0	1.9	1.9		0.9	61	60	30	8	
Oceania	**3.2**	**2.5**	**2.4**	**2.2**		**1.1**	**67**	**37**	**30**	**23**	
Australia/New Zealand	**2.6**	**1.9**	**1.9**	**1.8**		**0.9**	**52**	**23**	**17**	**12**	
Australia [21]	2.5	1.9	1.9	1.8		0.9	49	21	16	11	
New Zealand	2.8	2.1	2.1	1.9		1.0	65	33	25	19	
Melanesia	**5.8**	**4.5**	**3.7**	**3.1**		**1.6**	**123**	**68**	**54**	**44**	
Fiji	4.2	3.4	2.6	2.3		1.2	59	63	43	46	
New Caledonia	5.2	2.9	2.1	1.9		1.0	77	35	19	18	
Papua New Guinea	6.1	4.7	3.8	3.2		1.7	140	69	57	46	
Solomon Islands	7.2	5.5	4.1	3.3		1.8	142	85	54	33	
Vanuatu	6.1	4.8	3.4	2.9		1.6	86	70	45	36	
Micronesia	**5.3**	**3.7**	**2.8**	**2.5**		**1.3**	**85**	**68**	**30**	**17**	
Guam	4.1	2.9	2.4	2.1		1.2	93	78	50	41	
Kiribati	5.0	4.6	3.8	3.2		1.7	54	46	21	8	
Micronesia (Fed. States of)	6.9	4.8	3.3	2.7		1.5	75	48	19	7	
Polynesia [22]	**5.7**	**4.0**	**3.0**	**2.6**		**1.4**	**69**	**45**	**30**	**19**	
French Polynesia	4.9	3.1	2.1	1.9		1.0	96	57	38	28	
Samoa	7.0	4.9	4.2	3.5		1.9	62	34	28	16	
Tonga	5.5	4.6	3.8	3.2		1.8	31	26	17	11	

Notes:

The designations employed in this publication and the material presented in it do not imply the expression of any opinion whatsoever on the part of the Secretariat of the United Nations concerning the legal status of any country, territory, city or area or of its authorities, or concerning the delimitation of its frontiers or boundaries. The term "country" as used in the text of this report also refers, as appropriate, to territories or areas. The designations "more developed", "less developed" and "least developed" countries, areas or regions are intended for statistical convenience and do not necessarily express a judgement about the stage reached by a particular country or area in the developing process.

The tables and figures presented are from the medium variant of the World Population Prospects: The 2015 Revision, the official United Nations population estimates and projections prepared by the United Nations Population Division. Data are also available in digital form and can be consulted at the Population Division's web site at www.unpopulation.org. Users requiring the complete results of the 2015 Revision can purchase them on CD-ROM. A description of the data contained in the different CD-ROMs available and an order form are posted on the web site of the Population Division.

A minus sign (-) before a figure indicates a decrease.

A full stop (.) is used to indicate decimals.

Years given refer to 1 July.

Use of a hyphen (-) between years, for example, 1995-2000, signifies the full period involved, from 1 July of the first year to 1 July of the second year.

An em dash (—) indicates that the value is zero (magnitude zero).

A 0 or 0.0 indicates that the magnitude is not zero, but less than half of the unit employed.

Numbers and percentages in this table do not necessarily add to totals because of rounding.

(a) More developed regions comprise Europe, Northern America, Australia/New Zealand and Japan.

(b) Less developed regions comprise all regions of Africa, Asia (except Japan), Latin America and the Caribbean plus Melanesia, Micronesia and Polynesia.

(c) The group of least developed countries, as defined by the United Nations General Assembly in its resolutions (most recently, 68/18) included 48 countries in 2015: 34 in Africa, 9 in Asia, 4 in Oceania and one in Latin America and the Caribbean.

(d) Other less developed countries comprise the less developed regions excluding the least developed countries.

(e) The country classification by income level is based on 2014 GNI per capita from the World Bank.

(f) Sub-Saharan Africa refers to all of Africa except Northern Africa.

Country or area	Share of total fertility by women under age 20 (per cent) 2010-2015	Age-specific fertility rate 2010-2015 (births per thousand women in age group)							Age distribution
		15-19	20-24	25-29	30-34	35-39	40-44	45-49	
Northern America	8	28	81	106	98	48	10	1	
Canada	4	11	44	96	108	53	10	0	
United States of America	8	30	84	107	97	48	10	1	
Oceania	6	30	93	124	132	79	22	5	
Australia/New Zealand	4	17	56	102	125	71	15	1	
Australia [21]	4	16	53	102	126	72	15	1	
New Zealand	6	25	72	105	122	71	15	1	
Melanesia	7	54	178	178	148	104	48	22	
Fiji	8	43	158	141	94	58	22	5	
New Caledonia	5	19	97	121	97	65	27	1	
Papua New Guinea	7	57	183	182	155	111	53	27	
Solomon Islands	7	54	184	213	178	110	52	21	
Vanuatu	7	45	171	179	138	92	43	14	
Micronesia	5	30	113	169	151	76	25	4	
Guam	10	50	134	137	97	51	13	1	
Kiribati	3	21	119	216	228	127	39	8	
Micronesia (Fed. States of)	3	19	104	189	201	112	34	7	
Polynesia [22]	5	30	119	168	149	93	29	3	
French Polynesia	9	38	96	111	93	57	18	1	
Samoa	3	28	155	237	216	146	46	5	
Tonga	2	17	111	210	222	140	47	11	

(1) Including Agalega, Rodrigues and Saint Brandon.

(2) Including Zanzibar.

(3) For statistical purposes, the data for China do not include Hong Kong and Macao, Special Administrative Regions (SAR) of China, and Taiwan Province of China.

(4) As of 1 July 1997, Hong Kong became a Special Administrative Region (SAR) of China.

(5) As of 20 December 1999, Macao became a Special Administrative Region (SAR) of China.

(6) The regions Southern Asia and Central Asia are combined into South-Central Asia.

(7) Including Sabah and Sarawak.

(8) Including Nagorno-Karabakh.

(9) Refers to the whole country.

(10) Including Abkhazia and South Ossetia.

(11) Including East Jerusalem.

(12) Including Transnistria.

(13) Including Crimea.

(14) Refers to Guernsey, and Jersey.

(15) Including Åland Islands.

(16) Including Svalbard and Jan Mayen Islands.

(17) Including Kosovo.

(18) Including Canary Islands, Ceuta and Melilla.

(19) The former Yugoslav Republic of Macedonia.

(20) Including Saint-Barthélemy and Saint-Martin (French part).

(21) Including Christmas Island, Cocos (Keeling) Islands and Norfolk Island.

(22) Including Pitcairn.

ISBN 978-92-1-151542-8

15-15253